My Body My Temple

By

Carol K. Prill

ISBN: 978-1-4033-3954-6 (e)
ISBN: 978-1-4033-3955-3 (sc)

This book is printed on acid free paper.

Edited by Rhonda Wiczer Washer, M.S. in Ed., NCTMB

Rhonda received her Bachelors Degree from Northern IllinoisUniversity in 1972, and a Masters Degree in Education Administration in 1975. As a holistic consultant, educator and therapist, Rhonda has her own private practice called LifePath.®

1stBooks - rev. 12/14/12

*This book is dedicated
to my husband
Clarence E. Prill, D.C.
who patiently taught me how to
live a healthy lifestyle, and
persistently "walked the talk."*

Acknowledgements

To God be the glory for the marvelous creation of the human body. I thank Him for healing of mind, body, soul and spirit as He lead me to my resources.

I am grateful to my friend Eldyth Cristopher, who introduced me to the concept of detoxification, and for my mentor Mary Raistrick, who has dedicated her life to helping individuals stay well.

A special "thank you" is extended to my clients who shared their wisdom and experience as they traveled their journeys back to restored health.

I am indebted to the many authors who have written books sharing their knowledge of natural healing.

Abstract

The body is exposed daily to environmental chemicals and pollution. Diets contain additives, food coloring and flavoring to enhance the taste. Drinking water is filled with chemicals, as a result the body can acquire toxins followed by an illness. My Body, My Temple is a beginner's guide to detoxifying, rebuilding and maintaining a healthy body.

"Do you not know that you

Are the temple of God and that

The spirit of God dwells in you?"

The Bible 1 Corinthians 3:16

Table of Contents

Introduction

He that hath a truth and keeps it,
Keeps what not to him belongs.
But performs a selfish action,
And a fellow mortal wrongs.

Andrew Jackson Davis

A healthy mind and body is necessary for individuals to live optimally. All activities of living take on a positive nature when we are well and full of energy. It is taken for granted by many. Changes in an individual's health status may develop slowly and not exist as a problem until an illness manifests. A "wake-up" call may come in the form of an acute illness, chest pains, dizziness, depression or other discounted symptoms. The body's alarm system is not heeded. Nothing is checked out; no changes are made; and the body continues to perform the very best it can under the circumstances. Sooner or later, the body will become ill.

A beginner's guide to detoxification, rebuilding and maintaining a healthy body, explains why toxicity occurs, and what actions are needed to detoxify. Listening to the body is the first step, taking corrective action is the second.

My Body, My Temple is written to honor the body with respect for the wonderful activities it performs every minute of our lives. Keeping the body clean, nourished, spiritually nurtured and healthy is honorable to God. The body is God's temple.

Chapter One
Childhood Health

What do you remember about being sick as a child? You may not think it is relevant to reflect back on what your body experienced at a young age. You may question the impact on your life now. After all, during most of our childhood discomforts, we were told we would "outgrow it", or, we'll "get over it". This may have been true for many people, as young bodies have a marvelous way of compensating for injuries and insults. However, this is not true of everyone, and many adults are suffering from unresolved childhood health problems. There may be several reasons for this. The first, we are often afraid to tell our parents about not feeling well, having a pain, or problem because of the reaction it may invoke from them. Perhaps we were made to feel guilty if we created an inconvenience for someone else, such as mother missing work, or being unable to go on with her plans for the day. Perhaps our parents were unemployed with no means to pay for medical care. Another reason one may not report an illness or injury is because they may have been in forbidden territory when the injury occurred. It was not uncommon to hear, "that is what you get for not listening to me", which implies one deserves to be hurt, or they caused it. It would have been more appropriate to help the child see the relationship between their actions and the injury they received. Such insensitive comments send a strong message that the injury is not important, or that the child's feelings of pain are not important. The injury may not appear serious, but there may be lasting implications unknown at the time. I used to wonder why my mother become upset when my siblings or I become ill or injured. I thought the children should be upset, not the mother. Another reason for not expressing illness is fear of being discounted by parents, siblings, teachers or other significant people in our lives. Parents often view the expression of illness as a means of manipulation or to gain attention. Granted, as children we have probably experienced all of the above, and we did not understand how our illness or injury impacted the family. However, there are legitimate complaints from children that go unheeded and later develop into chronic conditions to be dealt with in adulthood.

Perhaps you have some unpleasant memories, as I do, about what went on in, with, and around my body as a child. Children are powerless over most activities in their lives. They have small bodies and can be picked up, carried, pushed and pulled where adults want them to be placed. Children are told when to eat, sleep, sit, talk and walk. Most adults would not be able to tolerate or process the amount of commands given a child in a day. Children are very special people, as you were as a child and as you are in adulthood.

Let me share with you some of the experiences of my childhood and how I believe they impacted my health as an adult. I am not judging parents or health providers. I am just observing what I experienced in childhood and some of the health problems that I had in the past and may still be challenged with today as an adult. It is also a review of how some perceived health problems were resolved, remembering that we perceive the world differently through the eyes of childhood.

Infancy and Early Childhood

One of my earliest memories is that of having dreams while still sleeping in my crib, where I imagined seeing worms hanging on the rails of the bed. I was terrified. I remember my mother comforting me and rocking me in a small rocking chair that now sits in my bedroom. When she recalled my childhood, she told me that I would sometime gag on what she thought were worms attempting to come up my throat. As an older child I remember seeing worms in the toilet, and I remember crying from stomach ache. One has to wonder where these critters come from at such a young age, in such a young body?

4

Usually parasites (worms) are transferred as eggs that hatch in a body where the conditions are conducive to their life cycles. They can be taken in the body by direct contact, or as eggs on fruits, vegetables and grains, and some through the air, such as the hookworm. (1)(Kroeger) Pinworms in children are common and transferred to others very easily. My siblings and I willingly shared the sand pile with our pet cats and dog named Wolfe. Once parasites have inhabited a body, the eggs can live in a dormant stage for years. Later when the conditions are met for them to hatch, the adults begin to multiply and create health problems in the body. Primarily, the parasites eat the good nutrients consumed, depriving the body of valuable vitamins and minerals. Secondly, the parasites discharge their toxic waste into the host, creating a disturbance in the internal environment of the body. This imbalance weakens the immune system, making the body vulnerable. Do not let anyone convince you that parasites are a third world problem and not of concern to people living in the most advanced country in the world. Parasites are a contributing factor to many health problems experienced by adults today. (2)(Clark) Having administered over 2,000 colon hydrotherapy sessions, I personally have seen parasites flushed from my clients and listened to numerous reports of improved health after clients have taken remedies for parasites. To this day, I continue to be challenged with parasites in my body.

With experience over the years, I am now alert to the beginning reoccurring symptoms and take measures to eliminate them. I am winning the battle!

As a preschooler I worried about my belly button sticking out. I was aware that the belly button on my sister and brother did not stick out like mine. I remember poking it down with my finger and being disappointed each time it would pop back out. However, to my knowledge I have not had any physical problems connected to this condition, but obviously as a small child I was emotionally preoccupied and self-conscious regarding this aspect of my body. A small hernia created by an undeveloped muscle was self-correcting, but to a small child it caused great concern. I remember asking my mother about it numerous times. She asked the country doctor about it in my presence to assure me that I was fine.

Other conditions of infancy that may continue into adulthood are problems created by fungus flourishing in the wrong places, or growing out of control. What is commonly known as "thrush" in the mouth is the result of candida albicans, a fungus, occurring in the wrong place in the body. Its natural place is in the intestines where it is instrumental in producing the amino acid methionine and a vitamin, biotin. (3)(Foley) It may be present in the vagina of the mother who delivers the infant, or it may be contracted from contaminated nipples on bottles. If thrush is temporarily suppressed with drugs, it can reoccur later in the child or in adulthood, as a chronic fungal infection and create numerous other health problems. (4)(Kaufman)

Childhood and Adolescence

Having sore feet is another problem I remember from childhood. Just about the time the new saddle shoes purchased for the start of the school year, were adequately broken in and comfortable to wear, it was time for summer vacation. Then next fall it was time for a new pair. To this day I cannot stand to wear tight or ill-fitting shoes.

Grieving, in children, is something that may not be recognized as a physical health problem at the time, but can create emotional and mental problems later in life. When I was ten years old, my infant sister died. My mother was ill for what seemed a long time. She remained hospitalized for a month with complications of a blood clot in her leg. When she returned home, our family was not the same, and my mother was never very well after that time. I am aware the sadness surrounding that time of my life impacted me emotionally, as a child and on into adulthood.

During the adolescent years when hormones were becoming active, my menstrual periods were very heavy. It was such an inconvenience to take supplies to school, and I was fearful that the flow would come through to my clothing. The country doctor treated me as having an iron deficiency and I would take the little green, triangular pills from time to time. I do not remember whether they made a significant difference.

As a teenager, I did not know about PMS (pre-menstrual syndrome), but I believe I would have met the requirements. However, mood swings are considered normal in adolescence, so this issue was never addressed.

Hormonal imbalances follow many female teenagers into womanhood, causing problems until it is decided that a hysterectomy is the only solution for the various symptoms. The hysterectomy then is the springboard for another series of problems, such as constipation, continued hormonal imbalances, and prolapse (falling down) of the bladder, vagina and colon.

As a child I had silver amalgam fillings containing mercury put into my teeth.

Shortly thereafter, I began having skin problems, little bumps appearing on my forehead and around my nose, but they would never come to a head or get red. They were just hard bumps under the skin. I remember the country doctor assuring my mother and I, that it was just teenage acne and would go away after giving birth to children. As an adult, after going to several dermatologist and being given various other diagnosis, I stopped searching for the answer. I was told, by one doctor, the only thing that could be done is to surgically incise each bump and remove the contents. So that is what I started doing with a needle. At times I created a bloody mess on my face! After reading information on metals and how they settle in the body, I am of the opinion that these bumps are filled with metal filled debris the body is sealing off to keep it out of the bloodstream. Mercury from the filling is not the only metal to cause concern. Aluminum cookware, soda cans, and aluminum foil are sources of aluminum toxicity. My mother had a set of aluminum cookware that prepared many delicious meals. Later my mother purchased a beautiful set of stainless steel cookware, only to learn years later that nickel is emitted from stainless steel. (5)(Foley) Two years ago a hair analysis revealed mercury, nickel and aluminum in my body, although I have worked diligently to remove these metals.

Later, in adulthood, I had braces put on my teeth. I then underwent an emergency abdominal surgery for the removal of a grapefruit sized tumor on my small intestine. During this surgery, a complete hysterectomy was also performed. My incision would not heal. I could not regain my strength and felt very sick, even though x-rays, an MRI and blood test indicated I was fine. The doctors insisted there were no complications and started me on hormone replacement therapy and an antidepressant. This protocol made me feel worse, not better. This was the beginning of my search for why I felt so sick. The quest for restored health led me to the alternate healing methods.

From what I was able to learn from reading and talking with my chiropractor, dentist and other natural health practitioners, it was concluded that mercury and possibly other metals had probably settled into the incisions and delayed the healing process. I believe braces moving old amalgam fillings released mercury into my bloodstream and carried it to the incision. Much information is available regarding the symptoms created from toxic levels of mercury in the body. My journey back to health led me to have seven fillings replaced with porcelain fillings and a root canal removed. My health continues to improve as I eliminate mercury and other metals from my body. My advise to parents is that they insist their children not receive amalgam fillings in their teeth.

There were other health issues as I grew up on the farm. A fall from a porch at a friend's home resulted in a broken collarbone. The country doctor wrapped it close to my body and it healed properly with no complications. However, not all children are so lucky. Often there are injuries to soft tissue, joints, backs, tailbones and extremities that go unreported to adults. The acute pain may subside, but the injury may remain. Over a period of time the sensation of pain may change due to increased pain tolerance and the nerve becomes less sensitive. Tissue may be injured with impaired nerve and/or blood flow. After a period of time the tissue weakens and bacteria, virus or fungus may settle in to create a toxic condition. This may go unnoticed, although a state of fatigue or chronic infection may be present and the child does not feel well. It is possible for the body to seal off a particular problem, in the attempt to protect the rest of the body. This condition may not create problems until later in adulthood, when an abscess, tumor or degenerative condition develops.

Reoccurring abscesses on my buttock was an embarrassing condition for me to experience. Many times I would not tell my mother when they were present, but there were times it was necessary for the country doctor to lance them. This was done without any local anesthesia. It was painful and so were the dressing changes. The worst part was not being able to go outside and do what I loved to do, such as ride on the tractor or my brother's pony. Knowing what I now know to be true, I apparently had a chronic infection in my body.

Children living in cities, especially large cities, encounter some of the same health challenges as those of us growing up on a farm. However, they encounter a different environment with it's own health hazards, such as busy streets, car fumes, crowded living conditions, and perhaps, more processed foods. Generally, children growing up on a farm usually have very wholesome diets with parents growing most of their own food, canning fruits and vegetables for the winter months, eating eggs from healthy, corn fed chickens and meat free from hormones and irradiation. Fast food restaurants were not an option. I was ten years old when we were on our way home from a family vacation, when I remember seeing my first famous hamburger stand selling hamburgers for fifteen cents.

Although I have no memory of respiratory problems, more and more children today have problems involving the respiratory system. This may be in the form of asthma, frequent colds, ear infections, bronchitis, viral infections and pneumonia.

Allergies often plague children, creating a need for special food and environmental requirements. This may be a financial burden on the family, creating additional stress at home. Food is a very important symbol of loving and nurturing children. When this has limitations and restrictions, parents may feel they are not being the good parent they want to be to their child. Real or imagined guilt only adds to the already stressful situation.

Trauma

The cells in the body contain the physical structure, the intelligence and the spiritual nature that connects us to God. The body is not composed of isolated parts. Intelligence is not located only in the brain, but each cell has the capacity to act intelligently and to communicate with other cells in the body. When we hurt a toe, the whole body is affected. Pain is registered in all cells, not just the injured toe.

There are three classifications of trauma to the human body. (6)(Stephenson) The three types of trauma are physical, chemical and emotional. When physical trauma occurs, it is obvious; it may be a bump on the head, a cut on the leg or a broken bone. We can identify the injury, express the pain and find a treatment to mend the damage. In chemical trauma, the body chemistry, or (homeostasis) chemical balance is effected and becomes unbalanced. If the body is not able to regain its balance and the condition continues, a toxic condition can develop in the body. Examples of chemical trauma are: poor food choices that are not assimilated in the body, some medications, street drugs, tobacco, pesticides, and household cleaning products. Emotional trauma is that which is not in harmony with the spiritual nature of the cell. The human body was made by God to be a vessel for positive vibrations. Thoughts travel from one cell to another by vibration.

Speech travels from one person to another by vibration. When the human body encounters negative thoughts from either internal sources, such as the individuals thoughts, or from external sources, such as other people's words or actions, they are registered in the cell. The vibration will have either a positive or negative impact on the cell. A positive vibration traveling from cell to cell strengthens the immune system. A negative vibration creates a chemical imbalance that suppresses the immune system. When the immune system is suppressed, it open the door to illness.

When illness is present in the body over an extended period of time, physical characteristics may also change. Actually, if any one of the three causes of trauma occur, ultimately, all three will be involved.

Abuse of any kind, whether it is verbal, sexual, emotional or physical, is a great insult to the body, mind and soul of an individual. Children are very vulnerable to abuse, since they are not equipped, or in some situations, not allowed to protect themselves. They often cannot maintain outward composure or internal balance, leading to behavior problems, which result in more abuse. Sooner or later, there is risk for illness of some nature to manifest, since the stress of abuse depresses the immune system. Often, adults, who were abused as children, are not aware of the connection between the abuse and their current health status.

Think back on your childhood to see if you can identify health problems that perhaps were not addressed. Are any of them still present? It is not to late to start the journey back to health. Let's get started!

Chapter Two

Fasting

The human body is composed primarily of water and minerals, in addition to protein, fat, and vitamins. The first step in the detoxification process is to reduce nutritional needs to bare essentials for a short period of time. Since the most basic need in the body is water, that is all that is consumed for approximately three days. This is called fasting. Fasting enables the body to burn up and eliminate waste from the cells.(7)(Walker) For detoxifying purposes, use distilled water, water without minerals. This will pull out toxins and some minerals, called electrolytes, from the body tissues. Although there are commercially prepared products that have electrolytes in the water, for the purpose of detoxification, pure water is used. If distilled water is not available, filtered water is used.

During detoxification, toxins are pulled from muscles and other tissues and deposited into the bloodstream for elimination. Headaches and fatigue (feeling tired and weak) may occur. One-fourth teaspoon sea salt dissolved in four ounces of water may bring some relief. Sea salt contains basic minerals required by man, especially sodium chloride which constitutes approximately 55 per cent of its composition. Chlorine's function is to cleanse the toxins from the body.(8)(Batmanghelidj)) Sea salt can be purchased at a health food store. It appears brown or gray in color, with a tendency to clump. Commercial salt is white with additives that prevent it from clumping

Drink at least four ounces of water every one half hour and when you become thirsty. Drinking large amounts of water at a time has no special advantage, since that practice may drain off needed nutrients. Do not wake yourself to drink water through the night. However, if you are up to eliminate, drink water again. Different body types and structures will have different water requirements. The average length of a fast is two or three days. Some people may not be able to tolerate the discomfort, yet others can fast for longer periods. Do not go beyond five days on a fast. The body may tolerate it at the present moment, but during the fast, the body is using its reserve supply of elements and prolonged fasting depletes the supply needed for future use. It is best to fast when you are not required to work or be around other people. You may become weak and need to rest, or you may become irritable and not very pleasant to be around. While fasting you may experience headaches, rashes, weakness and fatigue

Modifications of a water fast can be found in numerous books on natural health. Choose the diet that is going to best suit your needs. The water and salt fast should be safe for most individuals who do not have an existing medical condition that would inhibit them from fasting.

Each cell is similar to a small factory. Products go in; products are used by the cell to make energy, and then the waste products leave the factory. During the fast, only water is entering to bath the cell. The cell can rest, allowing the water to do its cleansing work, carrying the waste into the bloodstream. As each cell eliminates waste products into the bloodstream, they are carried to the four organs of elimination: skin, lungs, kidneys and colon. If the organs of elimination are on overload, some of the toxic "wash water" from the cells will stay in the bloodstream, creating a condition known as autointoxication, meaning you are absorbing your own toxins. Some of the symptoms created by autointoxication are: headaches, acne, stiffness, generalized aching all over and fatigue. The goal is to remove these toxins from the body as soon as possible.

Clients seeking detoxification, have two options, the slow track or the fast track. The slow track may be necessary for some clients who are very weak and ill. They may need a period of rebuilding the body before they start to detoxify. This is done with herbs, special diets and food supplements. Other clients who appear to be healthy, yet desire to feel better through detoxification, often choose the fast track, which includes colon hydrotherapy or self-administered enemas, in addition to herbs, a special diet and whole food supplements. Instructions for a self administered enema is in the appendix. Colon hydrotherapy sessions are administered by a professional healthcare provider. An enema or colon hydrotherapy session is recommended during and after a fast to eliminate the toxins from the body.

Chapter Three
Elimination

It is vitally important to keep the four organs of elimination open, to dispose waste from the cells. A brief review of each organ explains its importance in maintaining a strong immune system for a healthy body.

SKIN

The skin is a large organ composed of five layers of cells covering the body. Supporting the surface layers of cells is connective tissue with fibers, blood vessels, nerves, lymph vessels, hair follicles and sweat glands. The skin continually receives circulating blood to cells bringing nutrients, and secretes sweat from glands and oil from hair follicles.

The skin plays a vital role in regulating the body temperature via the sweat glands. Brain centers detect when the blood temperature is elevated and initiate activity in the sweat glands. Sweat is composed of the same inorganic components as blood, only in lower concentrations. The primary salt is sodium chloride. Organic components of sweat includes urea, uric acid, amino acids, ammonia, sugar, lactic acid and ascorbic acid and water. As the warm sweat leaves the gland, water evaporates taking the heat with it; thus, sweating helps to lower the body temperature. Heat is also lost from the body as the blood vessels dilate allowing more blood to come to the surface for evaporation. Sweat is almost odorless. Odor is produced by the combination of sweat and bacteria on the skin. Hair follicles contain sebaceous glands that produce the oily substance, called sebum used to lubricate the skin.(9)(Guyton)

The skin functions to protect the body by its ability to detect sensations of pain, touch, temperature and pressure as the nerve impulses relay the message to the brain. By nature, the skin is elastic and serves as a protective covering with its ability to prevent passage of harmful physical and chemical agents into the body, while it inhibits excessive loss of water and minerals (electrolytes). The acid surface of the skin prohibits the growth of some bacteria, and is our first line of defense to protect the immune system.

Since the skin so wonderfully protects us from the outside, holds our body together, and regulates our internal environment, it is wise to provide excellent skin care and maintain its integrity. Keeping our internal environment, such as the bloodstream, free from unnecessary toxins and waste, makes it easier for the skin to secrete what is unnecessary and to retain what is needed. Sweat glands and hair follicles must be free to eliminate toxins. Applying soap, shampoos, cosmetics and lotions made from harmful chemicals to the skin deplete its natural oil supply, creating dry skin. Chemicals alter the skin's naturally acid surface, hindering it's ability to fight infection. Antibacterial soap is not a substitute for the skin's natural ability to protect against bacteria. Gases and volatile substances, such as pesticides and sprays, exposed to the skin are absorbed by the bloodstream and carried throughout the body. Long periods of sun exposure dehydrate the skin; while short periods of sun exposure increases blood flow to the skin's surface, facilitating detoxification.

The surface of the skin must be kept clean for it to function optimally. Using a dry brush on the skin stimulates new cell growth. The outermost layer of skin is shedding continuously and replacing dead cells with new ones. Non-toxic soap and shampoo keep the pores open for elimination and lubrication. Methods of detoxification through the skin include: soaking in water with sea salt, baking soda and/or epsom salt; and soaking in water containing herbal teas, tinctures or extracts, and essential oils. Exercise that produces sweat in the body keeps the sweat glands open and eliminates toxins with the sweat. Saunas heat the body to temperatures that increase blood flow and eliminate toxins through the sweat glands and capillaries close to the surface of the skin.

LUNGS

The lungs are cone-shaped organs which completely fill the front cavity of the body. Lung tissue appears as a spongy mass, starting out pink in color during infancy, and as dust, smoke and foreign materials collect in the lymphatic vessels surrounding the lung tissue, it becomes blue-gray in color during adulthood. The lungs appear as two inverted trees with the trunk of each attached to the trachea, or what is commonly known as the windpipe. The inhaled air makes it's way down the tree trunk (bronchi) to smaller limbs on the tree (bronchioles) and finally to the leaves (alveoli). The exchange of oxygen and carbon dioxide takes place only in the alveolar sac, which is surrounded by capillaries.

The interior of the lung is the most extensive body surface in contact with the environment. Whatever is inhaled, is in direct contact with the inner lining of the lung. The lining of the bronchial tube is composed of ciliated epithelium, cilia meaning hair like cells, and epithelium referring to outer layer of cells. Mucus is produced by the lining of the lungs. Cilia move back and forth to evenly distribute the mucus through the lungs, and constantly sweep out solids that accumulate. It is important that this lining be protected from aerosol spray, pollution, dust, and smoke so the flow of air through the lungs is easy and unobstructed, allowing the cilia to move freely. When we exhale, the lung expels toxic gases that were carried by the blood to the air sacs.

Formaldehyde gas commonly found in new mattresses, flame-retardant chemicals on children's sleepware, and new carpet is toxic when inhaled into the lungs. Dr. Theresa Warner, D.C. warns parents of the potential health hazards when small levels (0.1 parts per million) of formaldehyde are inhaled, over a period of time, creating what she calls "toxic sleep". These health problems are: headaches, dizziness, scratchy eyes and throat, nasal congestion, coughing and immune system abnormalities. (9 A)(Warner)

In a normal sized adult the internal surface area of the lungs is approximately the size of a tennis court. Normal life processes require about one square meter (meter= 39.3 inches) of lung surface for each kilogram (kilogram=2.2 pounds) of body weight. Consider then, the increased effort required of an obese person, to breathe, exchanging oxygen and carbon dioxide. When the surface area of the lungs is fixed, with increased need per body weight, more frequent respirations put additional stress on the heart. (10)(Guyton)

Cleansing the lungs of accumulated smoke, pollution and dust can be accomplished with the ingestion of herbs and aromatherapy. Natural health professionals can help you select the best herbs for your individual needs. Maintaining a suitable body weight for your body frame is important to conserve energy required for breathing. Exercise facilitates cleansing the lungs by producing body heat that liquefies bronchial secretions, moving inhaled foreign substance and accumulated mucus, up the trachea, to the throat and out the mouth.

KIDNEYS

The urinary system consists of two kidneys, which produce urine; two ureters, which convey urine to the bladder; and the urethra, which discharges urine from the bladder. The kidneys are bean-shaped organs located just above the waistline and slightly to the back of the body. The kidneys act as organs for clearing blood plasma of substances not needed by the body and keeping those required. Excretion and absorption of water, sodium, bicarbonate, chloride, calcium, magnesium and phosphate in the blood, are regulated by the kidneys. One fourth of the total blood volume passes through the kidneys every minute. This activity produces approximately six cups of urine daily. Urine is 90% water, in which salts, toxins, pigments, hormones, and waste from protein metabolism are dissolved. Again we see the significance of keeping our bloodstream free from toxic waste, since added stress can be placed on the kidneys, when cleansing increased toxins from the blood.

COLON

The two primary functions of the large intestine, also called colon or bowel, is to absorb water and minerals (electrolytes) into the blood stream and store fecal matter until it can be expelled. After digested food travels through the small intestine, and all the nutrients are absorbed, the remaining liquid contents empty into the large intestine via the ileocecal valve. This valve keeps the contents from flowing backward into the small intestine. The liquid contents, called chyme, travels through the large intestine, where water and some minerals, enter the blood stream by absorption through the colon wall.

Numerous bacteria inhabit the colon, commonly referred to as "good bacteria". Bacteria are capable of digesting cellulose from foods that supply negligible amounts of energy. The primary importance of bacterial activity in the colon is the production of vitamin K, vitamin B12, thiamin, riboflavin, and various gases that contribute to flatus (gas).

The colon wall absorbs large amounts of sodium and chloride. The mucosa of the colon secretes bicarbonate that helps neutralize the acid end products of bacterial action in the colon. Small openings on the surface of the colon wall secrete mucus that assist in moving the fecal matter through the colon. Nerves in the abdominal tissues, initiate impulses, causing the muscles within the wall to contract and move the contents through the colon. Constipation may occur if mucus gland like structures called crypts, become clogged with dried mucus, bacteria or fecal matter; if parasitic activity exists; or if the nerve supply is impaired by physical obstruction, chemicals, or metal toxicity.

Supporting the lining of the colon, called mucosa, is a layer of connective tissue, rich in cells capable of protecting the body against infection. These cells are lymphoid cells, lymphatic nodules, plasma cells, special white blood cells and macrophages, that circulate in the body ingesting microorganisms (bacteria), foreign particles or other cells.(11)(Weiss)

Lymphatic nodules, composed of lymphoid cells, are also embedded in connective tissue. Lymphoid cells are instrumental in the production of antibodies, the part of the blood the counteracts growth and harmful action of bacteria. Tiny blood vessels, called capillaries, collect fluid from tissue, that empties into lymphatic vessels, with one way valves that force the fluid into the nodules. Lymph is a clear liquid containing large numbers of white blood cells, a few platelets and red blood cells. As lymph passes through the nodules, or nodes, they filter bacteria from lymph before it goes into the blood stream. The colon's lymphatic system helps fight infection, with its supply of bacteria fighting cells, and the filtering process of the nodules.(12)(Jacob)

Lymph that contains digested fat absorbed in the small intestine appears milky. Too much fat can create congestion in the lymphatic system. Lymph is carried by vessels to the thoracic (chest) cavity where it empties into the bloodstream, and transported back to the heart. It is important that lymph be as clean as possible, to protect the heart from any unwanted bacteria. It is necessary to keep the lymphatic system flowing freely, since stagnation of any body fluids provides a place for parasites, bacteria, virus and fungus to grow. The body keeps lymph moving by producing new lymph and pushing old lymph forward. Pulsating arteries produce a massaging effect on lymph vessels, peristaltic contractions of smooth muscle in the intestine, and massaging action of the skeletal muscles on the lymph vessels, also keep the lymph flowing. Exercising the body is an excellent way to keep the lymphatic system moving and functioning effectively.

Blood vessels surrounding the colon, carry blood that has absorbed water and minerals from the colon, directly to the liver. The absorbed water also contains bacteria and toxins from the colon. The liver, must filter the blood, making it useable for the rest of the body. If the colon walls are encrusted with dried mucus, fecal matter and unfriendly bacteria, the water absorbed into the bloodstream will be toxic, placing an additional burden on the liver.

Discharge from the colon is feces (bowel movement), consisting of materials such as mucus, water, minerals and bacteria, not absorbed by the small and large intestine. The odor results from the compounds produced by the bacteria. These compounds are phenol, hydrogen sulfide, indol, skatole and ammonia.(13) (Hole) Years ago the Royal Society in Great Britain reported on the condition of auto-intoxication, which is the reabsorption of these toxins into the body, creating a variety of symptoms and illnesses. These conditions were reported to be: elevated blood pressure from tryptophan, headache, racing heart beat, depression from the accumulation of histamine, circulation problems, muscle irritation, liver and kidney problems from excessive phenol, and congestion in the body from hydrogen sulfide. Symptoms of a toxic colon and autointoxication are bad breath, as the body expels toxins from the lungs, a coated tongue, sore joints, stiffness, fatigue, skin problems, and rashes. When these toxins and poisons reenter the blood stream, they create problems all over the body.(14) (Mantell) When these conditions are given a label, or diagnosis, medications are given to treat the symptoms. These chemical medications enter an already intoxicated body and can create further toxicity.

Constipation is common in Americans; so common, that few believe it is a problem. It is a subject that has a variety of definitions, and one that most people are uncomfortable discussing with anyone, even their physicians. Each individual establishes a pattern of elimination that seems normal to them, and aren't aware that it may be the cause of other health problems they are experiencing. Natural health consultants teach that the human body should have the urge to eliminate after each sizeable meal. With the exception of physicians who specialize in digestive tract disorders, many medical doctors reassure patients that one or two stools a week is sufficient. Passing stools on a daily basis is no guarantee that the walls of the colon are free from parasites, impacted fecal matter and layers of mucus. Stools expelled from the colon should be formed, soft, easily expelled and brown in color.(15)(Walker)

The colon is very close to the reproductive organs in both males and females, allowing the transfer of toxins to these organs. Keeping the lymphatic and circulatory systems clean and open is vital to maintaining healthy tissues of the reproductive organs. Clients have reported improved sexual performance after receiving colon hydrotherapy.

The liver is not considered one of the organs of elimination, but it is essential for the detoxification process. About four and one half cups of blood enter the liver every minute, to be filtered and altered for further use. About one and one fourth cup of clean blood comes to the liver, to bring nutrition to the connective tissues and bile ducts within the liver. The liver is a large expandable organ capable of acting as a valuable blood reservoir in time of excess blood and storing it for future use when needed.

Kupffer cells are large phagocytes (cells ingesting bacteria, other cells and foreign particles) lining the sinuses (cavities) of the liver. Special high- speed motion pictures of the action of Kupffer cells, have demonstrated that these cells can cleanse the blood extremely well. Upon contact with a Kupffer cell, a bacterium is engulfed within 0.01 second and held until it is digested. Not over 1 per cent of the bacteria entering the liver, from the absorbed water from the colon, succeeds in passing through the liver.(16)(Guyton) We would lighten the load of the liver, if we could maintained a healthy colon, and take measures to keep it cleansed of toxins and bacteria.

Bile ducts, in the liver, carry bile produced by the liver, to the gallbladder, where it is stored for release when needed to breakdown fats in the diet. Bile salts are contained in the bile. Cholesterol is also made in the liver and released with the bile. The function of bile salts, in the bile, is to keep cholesterol in a liquid state. Cholesterol is needed for the formation of hormones, cortisol and progesterone. Cholesterol not used by the body is reabsorbed, carried back to the liver to do its work and is excreted.

Cleansing the liver is important. Bile ducts can become congested and plugged with bile thickened with cholesterol. One of the most effective methods of cleansing the liver and gallbladder, naturally with food, is found in the writings of Hulda Clark, in *The Cure for All Diseases.* Gallbladder problems often are eliminated with the practice of liver cleansing, possibly avoiding the necessity for surgery. If the gallbladder is removed, the problems which created the gallbladder dysfunction continue to be present in the liver.

Therefore, cleansing the liver improves the function of both the liver and gallbladder. (16 A)(Jacob)

Chapter Four

Detoxify

The word detoxify is commonly used to identify the process of extracting toxins, which is commonly thought of as being limited to alcohol or drugs. The dictionary uses the words poisons and toxins interchangeably, as any substance that kills or injures when introduced into a living organism. In this book the term toxic will refer to any food, substance or environmental vibration which can injure cells of the body. With this definition, it is easy to see that toxicity can apply to most of the general population. So, when speaking of detoxifying, the focus is on removing anything that enters the body, or acts upon the body to impair its function in any way. If it is detrimental to the body, it is a poison, and the body has some degree of toxicity.

There has been an increased awareness of the toxicity in the environment. We are breathing the contaminates, drinking water with chemicals, eating food that has been grown with chemical fertilizers, eating irradiated meats from the grocery store, and covering our bodies with soap, shampoos and lotions made from chemicals. Pollution is very hard to escape, and it effects every aspect of life.

Symptoms of a toxic body are not the same for all individuals. What may be toxic to one person, may not be to another. However, there are common symptoms that can be generalized for many, such as rashes, offensive body odor, smelly feet, bad breath, headache, fatigue, foggy thinking, depression and restlessness.

We become toxic at the cellular level, and the process may be so slow we are not aware of what is happening. Then suddenly, one day we realize we "just don't feel right"; we have lost our desire, and are unable to do activities we once loved doing. We may not be acutely ill. We still function at our work, go through the daily routine and return home again, completely exhausted. Most people do not recognize this as an indication that something is hindering the body from performing optimally. In simple terms, the body is on overload! It simply cannot continue to process all the toxins it encounters and eliminate them from the body. This overload may be on the physical, mental and/or emotional level.

The cell is the basic unit of any organ. The health of the entire organ is no healthier then the weakest cell. It may seem that toxins in one little cell can't be all that important, since organs are made up of millions of cells. How can one apple, or potato effect the whole peck? Walk into a warm room where a rotting potato is deeply hidden in a sack; dig through the sack and see how many other potatoes are also beginning to rot. So it is with our cells. When one cell begins to deteriorate, it effects each cell around it, until the whole organ is affected. The process may be very slow, as illness develops gradually over a period of time; or the process may appear suddenly as an acute illness.

Cells become toxic when they are unable to function in the manner for which they were designed. Left alone, in the proper environment, the individual cell maintains itself, when provided with the required nutrients. It can repair, maintain and reproduce itself.

The body totally duplicates itself every three to five years. Some organs are faster than others. Studies have shown, for example, that red blood cells replenish themselves every twenty-eight days; while we regenerate our liver cells over a six-month period. For regeneration of organs to occur, the following four primary conditions for cell life must be met: nutrition, energy, elimination and reproduction.(17)(Northrup)

NUTRITION

Proper nutrition to the cells is vitally important. Most of us become weary hearing what we should eat, how much and at what time. We also become confused with conflicting reports about our foods. Our eating habits are considered a very personal and private affair, and we don't like anyone critiquing what we consume. I must confess that I fall in this category. I reluctantly analyze what I eat and how it is going to effect my body.

Two primary causes of poor health are incomplete digestion and a weak immune system, which create a cycle and effect each other. The body can make some vitamins, when proper nutrition is consumed. If protein and other nutrients aren't eaten, the body cannot keep the immune system healthy.(18) (Biser) Protein is of vital importance since it is the basic material of all living cells. The word comes from the Greek word "protos", meaning "first". The first thing the body needs is protein. (19) (Champe) The stomach produces hydrogen chloride to assist the enzymes as they break down protein into amino acids. Amino acids are used by the body to build the protein it needs. Many people with digestive problems are seen by a medical doctor and considered to have too much hydrogen chloride in their stomachs, but often, they do not have enough. Many times, simple digestive problems are diminished by drinking small amounts of undistilled apple cider vinegar in a glass of water, before eating protein. Apple cider vinegar is similar to the chemicals found naturally in the stomach.(20) (Clark) Many companies produce products that contain digestive enzymes and betaine hydrochloride (HCL) to facilitate the digestive process.

If the human body cannot digest, absorb or convert nutrients to energy, a toxic condition develops within the cells. Cellular activity produces waste within the cell that must be deposited into the bloodstream and eventually eliminated from the body. A build-up of toxic waste in the bloodstream can produce symptoms in the body, as mentioned earlier, and eventually causes disease and illness in various organs.

ENERGY

The process of eating, absorbing and assimilating what is eaten provides cell energy for growth and reproduction. However, there is another cell energy, I refer to as life energy, spiritual energy or universal energy, originating from God. This is the energy that is released when the body has deteriorated to the point of death. This energy exists in all cells and is quickly carried from cell to cell by nerve fibers. When the flow of energy along nerve fibers is blocked, the basic life force to the cell is depleted and the cell immediately begins to be compromised, resulting in impaired function, and necrosis (tissue death). When the life force has been impaired for an extended period of time, stagnation and toxic conditions are produced in the cells, leading to disease and sickness.

How does this happen? Visualize a picture of the spinal column, with nerves passing through the spinal cord, connecting with major organs to supply them with vital energy. Nerve interference to these organs can occur if there is a subluxation in the spinal column. A subluxation is a spinal vertebra that has lost its proper functional relationship with the one above and/or the one below. This results in the muscles on one side of the spinal cord becoming tight, while the muscles on the other side become loose, or flaccid.

As a result, the proper movement of the vertebral motor unit is limited and the life force leading to vital organs is blocked. When the life force cannot reach the cells of the organ, the cells cannot function, and they become toxic. Other conditions which block the energy from organs are physical pressure, chemical toxins, emotional trauma and/or a combination of all.(21) (Prill)

ELIMINATION

Cells have a natural process for eliminating waste products. When nerve energy to the cell is blocked, the cells cannot receive nutrients and oxygen required for normal metabolism; neither can they adequately eliminate toxic waste products. The build up of toxic waste products within the cells and nerve circuits that supply the cells, creates chemicals which contribute to increased nerve interference. Toxic cells have difficulty maintaining their normal activities, and after a period of time they are unable to function properly. This results in a weakened immune system, setting the stage for disease.

The Federal Centers for Disease Control and Prevention conducted a study in 1999 regarding the problem of toxicity in humans. Blood and urine samples from 3,800 people revealed high levels of toxic chemicals commonly used by most individuals. The survey tested for twenty-seven toxic substances; thirteen heavy metals, including lead and mercury, six metabolites, revealing the presence of pesticides; cotnine; and seven phthalates, which are chemical plasticizers frequently found in industrial solvents, cosmetics, soap, haircare products and, surprisingly, baby pacifiers. Humans have become "walking, talking toxic waste sites".(22)(Lowy) Although the American Chemistry Counsel believes further toxicity research needs to be completed to determine potential health hazards of our chemical environment, it is not difficult to look at our own health problems, or the health status of our children to know that we are all effected by our chemical environment and lifestyle. Respiratory problems, allergies and digestive problems in adults and children have reached such magnitude that specialists and clinics address these problems exclusively.

The effects of toxins on brain and nerve cells, organs, glands and muscles can intensify further from emotionally produced toxins, the ingestion of various drugs, (prescription and over the counter), street drugs, various heavy metals and poor nutrition. Poor eating habits can create autointoxication from the colon as a result of putrefaction from undigested foods in the colon and digestive tract. Autointoxication occurs when the body reabsorbs the toxins that should have been eliminated from the body.

REPRODUCTION

Cells need proper conditions and nutrients to reproduce. Hormones are an important component in the reproduction of cells. The liver is the organ that constantly monitors the need for specific hormones. As mentioned earlier, the body reproduces its organs every three to five years. Therefore, improvement in the health of the body, can be accomplished, by cleaning out the toxins, repairing damaged cells and reproducing healthy ones. Having said all this, do you now understand the importance of detoxifying your body? If you keep the cells clean, provide them with the food, water and environment they need; then they will take care of you!

Chapter Five

Rebuilding and Maintaining a Healthy Body

"Let's make our foods be our medicine
and our medicines be our food".
Dr. John R. Christopher

Rebuilding

The kind of food we eat and the amount consumed must be sufficient to supply the metabolic needs of the body, yet not cause obesity. The basic elements needed by the cells

49

for survival and reproduction are water, minerals, fats, carbohydrates and proteins. Roughly speaking, sixty-three percent of the body is water, twenty-two percent is protein, thirteen percent is fat and two percent are minerals and vitamins. (23)(Holford) Different foods contain different proportions of proteins, carbohydrates, and fats, which must be balanced so all segments of the body's metabolic systems are supplied with required materials.

Foods provide energy measured in calories. One gram of carbohydrates provides four calories of physiologically available energy for the body; fat provides nine and protein provides four. To make this energy available to cells, it must undergo further chemical reactions with the systems responsible for these physiological functions, through special cellular enzymes and energy transfer systems. When the energy from food combines with oxygen in the cells, large amounts of energy expressed as free energy is released.(24) (Guyton) Average Americans receive approximately fifteen percent of their energy from protein, about forty percent from fat and forty-five percent from carbohydrates. "Factors which determine the amount of energy (calories) the individual body requires are: sex, with women needing fewer calories than men; age, with older adults requiring less than adolescents and young adults; body structure, and level of activity".(25) (Ursell) Pregnant and lactating women have additional nutritional needs.

Protein

The body requires about 30 grams of protein daily to provide the essential amino acids necessary for building body tissue. Complete proteins in the diet are those having compositions of amino acids in appropriate proportions to each other, so that all the amino acids can be properly used by the body. Amino acids are the building blocks that are used to form structural proteins, enzymes, genes, proteins that transport oxygen, proteins of the muscle that causes contraction, and other activities both inside and outside each individual cell. Protein is needed in the diet to provide essential amino acids, but too much protein in the diet may also create problems. Once the cells are filled with all the amino acids they can use, the excess must be used as energy or stored as fat. This complex biochemical activity takes place in the liver, converting the ammonia released from the breakdown of protein, into urea that can be eliminated from the blood through the urine and sweat glands. Once again, the organs of elimination are important as they keep the body balanced, by discarding the excess products that accumulate in the blood.(26) (Guyton)

Carbohydrates

Carbohydrates function in the body to provide energy and to facilitate intercellular communication as part of the cell wall membrane.(27) (Champe) Carbohydrates should account for two-thirds of the total calories consumed daily. Carbohydrates are classified as "complex" (starches) or "simple"(sugars). Most of the simple sugars are "fast releasing", which means they raise the blood sugar quickly. However, in raw fruit, fructose is "slow-releasing.(28)(Holford) Simple carbohydrates, glucose and fructose, taste sweet, form crystals and dissolve in water. They are found in fruits, some vegetables and honey. Sugar can be processed from sugar beets and cane to create white table sugar. Glucose, also called blood sugar, is the most important carbohydrate in the blood. When reference is made to blood sugar levels, it means the glucose level in the blood. Complex carbohydrates are made up of many units of simple sugars, creating starches and many types of fiber.(29)(Ursell) Almost one half of all food eaten in one day, by the average American, is starch or sugar. Eating as much food in the raw form is preferred, since cooking and freezing alters the chemical properties of food, and diminishes its nutritional value.

Fats

The body's fat requirement, approximately forty-five percent of daily caloric consumption, may be visible in foods, such as butter or on a piece of meat, or they may be invisible, as in cheese, fried foods and cakes. Fats make food taste good, particularly when mixed with sugars in cakes and pastries. Fats are made up of fatty acids and are concentrated sources of energy. Fats are classified as saturated, monounsaturated or polyunsaturated, depending on the type of fatty acid that is present in the largest proportion. Certain fats consumed in reasonable amounts, are an essential part of a healthy diet. These fats are derived from plant and marine sources, such as nuts, seeds and fish, which contain monounsaturated fats.(30) (Ursell).

Water

Water comprises sixty-three percent of the body's entire composition. It is essential for many chemical activities to take place. Water is eliminated through the lungs, sweat and urine. It must be replaced each day through the consumption of foods and liquids. The body needs a minimum of forty-eight ounces (six cups) to sixty-four ounces (eight cups) of water a day. Exact needs depends on climate and levels of activity. For every hour of strenuous activity, add four cups water. Drinking water should be filtered.(31)(Ursell)

Maintaining a Healthy Body

Numerous books are available to provide information on food choices for maintaining a healthy body. Individuals may require special diets for medical reasons. Diets are designed to help individuals maintain, increase or decrease body weight. Diets are available to alter body chemistry and create undesirable living conditions for parasites, virus, bacteria and fungi. Special diets to detoxify the body must be followed by individuals, whose organs of elimination are compromised, or who are exposed to toxic elements on a daily basis. Healthy, chemically stable individuals are able to consume and assimilate average servings of a balanced diet.

Protect Your Body

Individuals are seldom informed of the risk of consuming foods that are readily available and popular. These foods produce toxins in the body and create conditions that put individuals at risk for physical diseases. A healthy body is maintained by avoiding certain foods, as well as knowing which foods should be eaten. Commonly popular foods that put the body at risk are: fried foods, which add additional fat for your body to metabolize, resulting in increased waste products in the bloodstream, soft drinks and artificial sweeteners, and bleached flour which contain chlorine that weakens the lining of the intestinal tract.

The following information on soft drinks taken from an article in *Townsend Letter of Doctors & Patients*, reports valuable information on how to protect you body. (32)(Field)

Soft drinks contain the following components: phosphoric acid, caffeine, sugar or aspartame or saccharin, caramel coloring, carbon dioxide and aluminum. These ingredients cause imbalances in body systems that result in debilitating diseases that show up after many years of abuse. These diseases have now become commonly thought of as "normal aging", when actually they are the result of destructive physiological consequences of ingesting soft drinks to contribute to "early aging" of the body.

Phosphoric Acid: *Soda contains phosphoric acid that taste sour. Sugar is added to make it taste good. Phosphoric acid is used to clean showers by dissolving minerals. A tooth will dissolve in it. The container warns that the acid is "harmful if swallowed". The body maintains a balance of it's calcium and phosphorus in the bloodstream in a correct combination for building new bones and remodeling old ones. The loss of calcium in the blood activates the parathyroid gland to secrete parathyroid hormone, which causes a release of calcium from the bone. When phosphorus from a soft drink enters the body, without a supply of calcium, the bloodstream balance is disturbed. Low level of calcium triggers another body system to* dissolve calcium from the bones, taken first from the spine and pelvic bones. In anticipation of more phosphorus entering the body, it over compensates and dissolves more calcium from the bone than immediately needed. The blood must now eliminate excess calcium; and it does so in the following ways: excretion in the urine, deposition in joints causing osteoarthritis, bursitis, gout, bone spurs bunions, kidney stones, and plaque in arteries.

Phosphoric acid is a strong acid that creates a decrease in the secretion of hydrochloric acid (HCL) necessary in the digestive process of fats and proteins. An important function of HCL is to stop the overgrowth of harmful bacteria, yeasts and parasites in the digestive tract.

Caffeine: Caffeine in soft drinks is an addictive drug that has the ability to stimulate mental alertness, overcome fatigue and enhance endurance. This stimulation is accompanied by constriction of cerebral arteries, rapid heartbeat, and high blood pressure. Caffeine is also a diuretic causing excessive excretion of urine. Adrenal exhaustion will result with repeated demands for adrenaline. Depriving caffeine users of their daily caffeine results in mental sluggishness, inability to think clearly, depression and a dull, generalized headache. Caffeine addiction is easy to deny and difficult to break because the long term effects are not immediately recognized.

Sugar: A 12-counce can of soda contains about 11 teaspoons sugar (one-fourth cup). Eating one-fourth cup sugar once or twice a day is empty food with no nutritional value. Sugar ingestion impairs kidney function, causing the excretion of calcium, magnesium, chromium, copper, zinc and sodium. The loss of calcium in the blood activates the parathyroid gland to secrete parathyroid hormone which causes the release of calcium from the bones. This results in osteoporosis, arthritis, bursitis and gout. Sugar in soda causes clumping of red blood cells impeding the delivery of oxygen and removal of carbon dioxide from the cells. This creates a buildup of waste in the body that accelerates aging and tissue toxicity. Sugar impairs immune function by hindering the white blood cell's ability to engulf and destroy bacteria. Sugar supports the growth of harmful bacterial and yeasts in the digestive tract. When food manufacturers advertise weight loss products as "fat free", but add sugar to the product to improve the taste, the body will convert the excess sugar into fat. This may be the reason that approximately fifty percent of the American people are overweight.

Aspartame, Saccharin and Caramel Coloring: If the soda is a diet soda, an artificial sweetener, aspartame replaces the sugar. When aspartame is digested, it breaks down into the following chemicals: aspartic acid, phenylalanine and methanol. Aspartic acid is an excitotoxin that can cause serious chronic neurological disorders. It can over stimulate neurons in the brain, to such an extent, that neurons are slowly destroyed before any obvious behavioral symptoms are noticed. Phenylalanine can cause decreased serotonin (a brain neurotransmitter related to emotion and sleep). Low serotonin levels lead to emotional disorders, depression or poor sleep quality. Methanol is metabolized into formaldehyde (a deadly neurotoxin and carcinogen) and formic acid (the active chemical in bee and ant stings). Methanol is a cumulative poison producing the following symptoms: headache, tinnitus (ringing in the ears), shooting pains, memory lapses, numbness and nerve inflammation. Saccharin and caramel coloring are considered to be carcinogens.

Carbon Dioxide and Aluminum: Soft drinks contain carbon dioxide. Carbon dioxide is a waste product that will need to be excreted by the lungs. Lining aluminum soda cans with plastic does not stop phosphoric acid from leaching (pulling out) toxic amounts of aluminum into the soda. Aluminum given to rats creates formations of tangled nerve fibers in brain tissue of the same type seen in brains of individuals who have Alzheimer's disease. Aluminum exposure increases the amount of bone breakdown, it also reduces the formation of new bone.

These beverages are replacing the water consumption required by the body, altering the body chemistry to such a degree as creating serious health problems. Schools, starting with nursery schools, now have vending machines with soft drinks readily available to growing children. The availability of soda machines found everywhere lures people to make unhealthy beverage choices.

In Summary, individuals need to listen to their bodies. When they experience discomfort, they need to become aware of what was eaten, and find natural solutions that do not result in further insult to the body. Health problems that have existed for years will not be resolved with three days of fasting and a colon cleanse. Lasting changes require lifestyle alterations. A toxic body requires a continued diet of raw, wholesome foods with limited starches and sugars. Clean, filtered water must be consumed on a regular basis, eliminating caffeine and sugar beverages. Change does not come easily when poor eating choices have been made for long periods of time. Young bodies can tolerate nutritional poor diets because of their adaptability; but in adulthood, the body becomes burdened with the results of continual, poor eating habits. Help children establish healthy food choices. It is a valuable gift, and will providing them with a lifetime of benefits.

Chapter Six
Healing With Prayer

Prayer is communion with God. To commune is to converse together intimately with someone. In prayer, it is conversing intimately with God. Talking intimately implies revealing information to another person that is not commonly shared. Prayer provides the opportunity to talk to God about issues we are unable or unwilling to share with other individuals.

Health problems are often kept secret out of fear. Fear immobilizes individuals to avoid seeking solutions to their health issues, as they imagine the consequences. They fear their vulnerability when ill or physically compromised. Individuals may believe they deserve to be ill as a result of wrong doing in their lives. When people do wrong, or do not follow God's will, they may believe God does not want to talk to them.

Prayer provides a safe haven for an individual's troubled spirit, since it is communicating with the creator who understands human behavior. In prayer the individual may talk intimately with God about the illness, sharing in detail the desire of the heart. Negative emotions of fear, anger, resentment and unforgiveness hinder the healing process. Prayer is therapeutic when deep hurts and negative emotions are released to God. We must become totally dependent upon God for His guidance in our journey back to restored health. When seeking answers to health challenges, God will provide them, and/or be a guide to the person who can help. The road back to health may be a jigsaw puzzle, finding one piece at a time until the whole picture is revealed. Becoming aware of God working in each small piece, increases gratitude for His mercy as He reveals solutions to health problems. Gratitude magnifies and enhances results far beyond expectations. Praise multiplies the energy available for healing, resulting in positive vibrations to stimulate the immune system.

Healing may be instant, it may require action on the part of the individual, or the results may come more slowly. Regardless of the prayer request, unanswered prayer provides the temptation for discouragement and disbelief in the power, goodness or willingness of God to act on our behalf. Finite (limited) minds cannot understand the infinite mind of God. We may never know "why" a specific prayer was not answered. Individuals in covenant (mutual and solemn agreement) with God, know that God is infinite, having all wisdom and knowledge, while they are not. The element of trust in a covenant provides the opportunity for acceptance of the unanswered prayer, believing a better solution will be provided in God's wisdom.

As a Christian, I believe healing energy is still active and available today, as demonstrated by Jesus Christ while He was on earth. He hears my prayers, and is my intercessor to God.

Prayer changes people and situations, and is available to you in this present moment, for your healing needs. There are many was to pray and have communion with God. The decision to pray for healing must come from the heart. God understands the language of emotions, and he hears the heart's desire.

Appendix

Self-Administered Colon Cleanse

The best way to cleanse the colon is to administer an enema. They may be self administered with the use of proper equipment, which can be purchased at a drug store at a reasonable price. Follow the directions for the correct assembly of bag and hose. In addition to the enema bag, you will need latex disposable gloves, paper towels and water-soluble lubricant.

Instructions for administering an enema was adapted from *Fundamentals of Nursing* by Taylor, Lillis and Lemone.(33)

Equipment
Enema set
Water-soluble lubricant
Solution
Disposable gloves

Temperature: warm to the inside of the arm.
For adult – 105° F-110° F (40° C-43 C)
For children – 100° F (37.7° C)

Amount:
Will vary depending on type of solution, age of the person, and the individual's ability to retain the solution. Average cleansing enema for an adult may range from six to eight cups.

Location

The location chosen for administration of the enema will be an individual preference. Lying in an empty bathtub with a towel for padding is recommended for individuals who have weak anal muscles and are concerned with leakage. However, this requires moving from the bathtub to the toilet to expel the contents after each fill into the colon. Another option is lying on the bathroom floor on a large towel. Place a plastic sheet or bag over the towel to protect the towel from leakage.

Solution

The solution for all enemas should be filtered, pure drinking or distilled water. Do not use unfiltered tap water.

Stimulating enema: One-fourth cup, freshly squeezed lemon juice, that has been strained, added to one enema bag. The lemon water facilitates removing encrusted mucus from the colon wall. Lemon juice provides vitamin C, potassium and calcium to the body through absorption by the colon wall.(Walker)

Maintenance enema: To maintain body temperature within normal range and to lower an elevated body temperature, one tablespoon sea salt may be added to the enema bag. The sea salt provides all the essential minerals, also called electrolytes, necessary for the body, as it is absorbed through the colon wall.

Special enema: Using teas or other solutions is a decision based on individual needs. One cup of chamomile tea to a bag of water may be useful as a sleep aid, to relieve pain and fever, to calm nerves and soothe rashes as it is absorbed into the colon wall.

Procedure

1.Assemble the necessary equipment. *Warm solution and check temperature with a thermometer or test on inner wrist.*

2.Wash your hands. *Clean hands stops the spread of germs.*

3.Add enema solution to the container. Release the clamp and allow fluid to progress through tube before reclamping. *Clear the air from the hose to prevent air from entering the colon.*

4.Administer the enema when you are free from interruption. *A relaxed environment facilitates a successful outcome.*

5.Put on disposable gloves. *Gloves protects the hands from germs in the feces.*

6.Elevate the solution to a level of 18 inches above the anus. *The container may be hung on a towel rack or special hook for this purpose. The fluid enters the intestine by gravity.*

7.Generously lubricate the hard end of the rectal tube for 2-3 inches. *Lubrication facilitates passage of the rectal tube through the anal sphincter and prevents injury to the lining of the rectum.*

8.Lie on the left side. Lift the buttock. Slowly and gently insert the rectal tube 3-4 inches. *Direct it at an angle pointing toward the belly button. Slowly insert the tube past the internal muscle to the anal canal that is approximately 1-2 inches in length*

9.If the tube meets resistance while inserting it, permit a small amount of solution to enter, withdraw the tube slightly, then continue to insert. Do not force entry of the tube. *Take several deep breaths to relax the* *colon muscles. Do not force the tube into the colon, as this may cause injury to the colon wall*

10.Once the rectal tube is inserted, release the clamp on the tubing and introduce the solution slowly over a period of 5-10 minutes, holding the tubing the whole time the solution is being instilled. *A slow flow of solution enables the colon to fill more effectively.*

11.Clamp the tubing or lower the container if the desire to defecate or cramping occurs. Take small, fast breaths. *Oxygen helps relax muscles and prevents the premature expulsion of the solution.*

12.After approximately one-third if the solution has been given, clamp the tubing and remove the rectal tube. *Retain the solution until the urge to empty in the toilet.*

13.Recommended, but not essential is the use of a small hand held massager moved in a clock-wise motion over the abdomen while expelling in the toilet. *This stimulates the intestinal wall and dislodges feces and gas.*

14.After expelling the contents of the colon, reinsert the rectal tube and repeat step 8. *This can be repeated as long as there are contents to be expelled. A second bag of solution may be necessary before the colon is totally empty.*

15. When complete, drain the bag and wash the rectal tube with a disinfectant. *Store in a dry place after allowing the water to drain from the bag and tube.*

*If the equipment is not properly cared for, abundant
bacteria in the colon can be spread.*

16.Remove disposable gloves and discard.

18. Wash hands thoroughly. *Washing hands stops the
spread of germs.*

A successful enema leaves a sensation of lightness,
emotionally as well as physically. The enema serves
several purposes: the removal of stored fecal matter and
accumulated gas, alteration of the ph of the colon to less
acid conditions, removal of encrusted mucus from the
colon wall, and the absorption of water into the body
with any additional nutrients that may had been added.

References

1

Kroeger, Hanna. (1191). *Parasites The Enemy Within.* Boulder, CO: Hanna Kroeger Publications.

2

Clark, Hulda Regher, PhD.., N.D. (1993). *The Cure for all Cancers.* Diego, CA: ProMotion Publishing.

3

Foley, March, D.C., N.D., (1997). *Integrating Your Wholeness.* East Moline, IL: The Universal Life Church.

4

Kaufman, Doug A., & Hunt, Beverly Thornhill (eds.) (2000) *The Fungus Link Rockwall, Texas:* MediaTrition.

5

Foley, Marcy, D.C., N.D., (1997). *Integrating Your Wholeness.* East Moline, IL: The Universal Life Church.

6

Stephenson, Ralph W., D.C., Ph.C. (1948). *Chiropractic Textbook.* Davenport, IA" Palmer School of Chiropractic.

7

Walker, N.W., D.Sc. (1949). *Become Younger.* Phoenix, AZ: Norwalk Press.

8

Batmanghelidj, F., M.D. (1997). *Your Body's Many Cries for Water.* Falls Church, VA:

9

Guyton, Arthur, C., M.D. (1976). *Textbook of Medical Physiology*. Philadelphia, PA: W.B. Saunders Company.

9A

Warner, Theresa, D.C., FICPA. (2001, December) "Children's Wellness: Toxic Sleep". *The Chiropractic Journal. p. 32.*

10

Guyton, Arthur C., M.D. (1976). *Textbook of Medical Physiology*. Philadelphia, PA: W.B. Saunders Company.

11

Weiss, Leon, M.D. (1988). *Cell and Tissue Biology*. Baltimore, M.D.: Urban & Schwarzenberg, Inc.

12

Jacob, Stanley W., M.D., F.A.C.S. $ Francone, Clarice Ashworth. (1970). *Structure and Function in Man*. Philadelphia, PA: W.B. Saunders Company.

13

Hole, John W., Jr. (1933). *Human Anatomy Physiology*. Dubuque, Iowa: Wm. C. Brown Publishers.

14

Mantell, Donald, J., M.D., (1986, May). "Colon Hydrotherapy and Its Clinical Applications." *The Nutrition and Dietary Consultant. 16-17.*

15

Walker, N.W., D.Sc. (1949). *Become Younger*. Phoenix, AZ: Norwalk Press.

16

Guyton, Arthur, C., M.D. (1976). *Textbook of Medical Physiology*. Philadelphia, PA: W.B. Saunders Company.

17

Northrup, Christine, M.D. (1998). *Woman's Bodies, Woman's Wisdom.* New York, N.Y.: Bantam Books.

18

Biser, Sam. (1995-1996). *Ancient Cleansing Formulas the Work-After Vitamins and Medicines Have Failed.* Charlottesville, Virginia: The University of Natural Healing, Inc.

19

Champe, Pamela C., Ph.D. & Harvey, Richard A., Ph.D. (1994). *Biochemistry.* Philadelphia, PA: J.B. Lippincott-Raven.

20

Clark, Hulda Regher, Ph.D., N.D. (1993). *The Cure for all Cancers.* Diego, CA: ProMotion Publishing.

21

Prill, Clarence E., D.C. (2001). *The Prill Chiropractic Spinal Analysis Technique.* Manuscript submitted for Publication.

22

Lowy, Joan. (2001, March 22). "Humans are 'walking, talking toxic waste sites'". *Journal Star, p. A3.*

23

Holford, Patrick. (1999) *The Optimum Nutrition Bible.* Freedom, CA: Crossing Press, Inc.

24

Guyton, Arthur C., M.D. (1976). Textbook of Medical Physiology. Philadelphia, PA: W.B. Saunders Company.

25

Ursell, Amamda. (2002). *Complete Guide to Healing Foods.* New York, NY: Dorling Kindersley Publishing, Inc.

26

Guyton, Arthur C., M.D. (1976). Textbook of Medical Physiology. Philadelphia, PA: W.B. Saunders Company.

27

Champe, Pamela C., Ph.D. & Harvey, Richard A., Ph.D. (1994). *Biochemistry.* Philadelphia, PA: J.B. Lippincott-Raven.

28

Holford, Patrick. (1999) *The Optimum Nutrition Bible.* Freedom, CA: Crossing Press, Inc.

29

Ursell, Amamda. (2002). *Complete Guide to Healing Foods.* New York, NY: Dorling Kindersley Publishing, Inc.

30

Ursell, Amamda. (2002). *Complete Guide to Healing Foods.* New York, NY: Dorling Kindersley Publishing, Inc.

31

Ursell, Amamda. (2002). *Complete Guide to Healing Foods.* New York, NY: Dorling Kindersley Publishing, Inc.

32

Field, Stan. (2002). The Curse of the Soft Drink. Townsend Letter for Doctors and Patients, Dec. 98.

33

Taylor, Carol, CSFN, RN, MSN, Lillis, Carol, RN, MSN, LeMone, Priscilla, RN, DSN. (1997). *Fundamentals of Nursing.* Philadelphia, PA: Lippincott-Raven.

The author may be located at the following address:

Natural Health Services

8804 W. Smithville Road

Mapleton, IL 61547

Phone: 309-697-5292

email: cknatural@insightbb.com